Diabetic Denial

The Family

Diabetic Denial

The Long Journey Home

Alexander Danny Joyeux

To order additional copies of this book, contact:
Xlibris
1-888-795-4274
www.Xlibris.com
Orders@Xlibris.com
772827

CONTENTS

RECIPES

Acknowledgments

I would like thank all who helped in my recovery and journey to a healthy beginning.

The Doctors, Nurses and Staff of Kaiser Permanent Hospital, Vallejo CA, their dedication to my health and recovery was vital to returning home and healing from such a traumatic experience. My neighbors whose concerns, gratitude and understanding gave me a sense of relief as guest crowded the area.

My family: Brothers and Sisters who supported me throughout my ordeal and continue   to show their love for me. My Cousins who accompanied me to all my medical appointments

To my Mother: Annette Joyeux a special thanks, as one does not understand love, until a mother gives it to you. My mother was the single most important person, who gave me the strength and will to fight back, to never give up.

To the many more not mention and know who they are, thank you for everything.

Cover Art work and Photography: FireSeason Studios, Oakland, CA

Dedication

This book is dedication to the millions of diabetic people around the world and the many more who are becoming aware as pre diabetics. I hope my story will aid in the awareness and commitment in combatting this issue. I want all to know you are not alone in this struggle, as it requires a lifetime of ups and downs in the pursuit of regulating a healthy lifestyle. Millions find it hard to combat and feel as though life dealt them some bad fate, but I am here to tell it was not so. I hope my story inspires you to make the changes that are necessary, so you can live a full productive and as natural a life as any other human being on the planet.

I also want to give a special thanks to my mother and family whose support gave me the strength and courage to continue on my journey. Family and friends can make all the difference in life, especially when we think; there is no one we can turn to. I found my strength through them and that carried me the rest of the way, it made all my convictions and determination that much more. Through their commitment to me, we were able to devise a dietary and quality of life plan; some of which I will share later in the reading. Our time on this planet should always be about making the best of what we have and how we can give to others, what we would want for ourselves. Which is why, I decided to share my personal experience, so many of you would not suffer the same fate.

May you read this short but honest story, of a man who was in denial, yet battled back to find comfort and a renewed calling to humanity!

"Diabetic Denial"

My name is Alexander D Joyeux and I have Type II Diabetes. Living with diabetes is difficult and a continual struggle.

When first diagnosed with Type 2 Diabetes in 2006, I went home and began over the next 6 months researching to gain a greater understanding. I immediately started exercising and testing my blood sugar on a daily basis, making sure my A1C was within the guidelines based on the research and doctors information. The results of exercise paid off right away, showing normal levels of sugar in my body, keeping sugars within the normal levels 80-110 or average of 93, life felt normal or I thought it was. I went back to my daily routine and thought nothing of it. Skipping appointments with my physician and of course; having my way with cake, ice cream and all other unhealthy snacks we loved as children.

I was in complete denial and, thought since I wasn't born with this disease, and had only acquired it through my excessive weight gain and unhealthy eating habits, usually at night consuming a big mac or two, with fries, and washing it down with an oversized coca coca cola, well my attitude was, I would be able to overcome and back to normal life, as if nothing happened, but that was not the case. Over the next 12 years, life was a roller coaster, I consistently battle with my sugars, graving for the sweet savory food and drinks would not allow me to walk away as one should and eventually it would have a life changing effect.

After a year of normal levels, I again went back to my old habits, binge eating and enjoying life. I would host backyard parties, attended endless other parties, with the food and drinks increasing at each event, and thinking life could not have been better. This was especially so when visiting my homeland, St Lucia; how I would just let loose, drinking 10 beers in 15 mins, eating plenty of island food heavy in carbs, but mostly consuming alcohol with its high sugar content. This lifestyle change the outcome of everything, as I now looked back on how it affected my health. health. The more I drank, the more I could feel pressure in my calves, at times becoming difficult to walk. Yet, it did nothing to slow me down. Then my feet started to swell almost daily. At first, I just blew it off as excess water, but the pain became more and more intense and what was every night, become every day and then every hour. I was ignoring the signs of a disease that was slowly taking over my body and life. Hey I was on vacation and at home, why let something that small stop a good thing. We all say this at some point in our lives; if I am walking breathing and enjoying the moment, why stop the fun, usually it gets us into trouble and so was the case. Upon wrapping up my vacation with family and assuring them I would make an appointment with my personal doctor once back home. Well as with many guys my age at the time, I just did not remember those promises. I stubbornly and blatantly ignored my doctor's calls and request to control my diet and increase exercise. Instead, I opted for more sugary drinks and bad carbs, which infected my body, while it was fighting to keep from further damage, to its internal organs. Time after time and day after day, high carbs and sugar found their way into my bloodstream; this decease began to get acquainted with other cells and disrupt normal body processes. To add more insult to injury,

I began working longer hours and getting less sleep, sometimes only 3-4 hour a night.

As an average American man with a family, working long hours became the norm in an ever changing competitive society. I focused on getting ahead in a world that was increasingly demanding more of our time and becoming more difficult to survive, sometimes 16-20 hours a day to keep up with an America that was leaving me behind, as with most middleclass Americans who saw the door to the dream growing further away and family losing out. I took on an iron man approach, ignoring the signs that presented it-self, such as; frequent urination, every 30 minutes. I chose to ignore my body; all the while it was being slowly destroyed. I chose to concentrate on being successful in my career and focusing on providing financial security for my daughters. Moreover, I enrolled in college to pursue a degree in IT management, dedicating every bit of energy I could generate to achieve a high order in education. I wanted to be a good role model for my daughters. I thought that by seeing my success in job and education, they would not have an excuse to strive or reach for the stars. It is called sacrifice and sometime it may require your life or some payment in exchange.

Life now; became a constant whirlwind of work and school, spending 16 hours at work and 4 hours attending school. My family rarely saw me and of course that part of my life started to derail. With my eyes on the task at hand, looking in the review mirror was not an option. As my family life began to fall apart, the disease started to take control, wanting more and more of my body and causing emotional changing experiences. My emotions and moods swung as in a terrible storm at sea; One day I am loving and calm, next day, I was angry and combative. Neither stopping to understand nor having the time to consider, I became more and more erratic and unbearable to live with. Home was a battleground and I found myself wanting to stay away, more and more. Opting for the good times with the guys and drinking. When not hanging with the guys, my job became a refuge. Finally, when the walls became too high to climb, my wife left, my family was in disarray and my health in declined.

On August 18, 2015, I returned from my second 2-month vacation, in St. Lucia, I simply just *lived it up*; Partying and drinking every day, having no care of this world, feeling free from the stress of the concrete jungle and dealing with the sudden death of a family member, who had pass in April. Upon returning from my vacation, it was back yet again to work and to daily life. After a month or so, I began to have slight pain under my left foot, telling no one of my health woes, keeping it to myself. As time went on, the pain become increasingly troubling to say the least, I sometimes had tears running down my face trying to maintain a workable composer, Pride; now was my worst enemy, more so than the pain or disease. Remembering the conversation I had with my good friend and work colleague, Francisco: about how I could no longer bare the pain nor was I able to stand on my feet. Yet; going to travel about two and a half hours to swap out a network card and how when completing this task, I would call and making an appointment to check on my foot. To this day I am not sure why I kept my word to do so, usually when I make an appointment, it was followed with a cancellation. Something divine stepped in, as with Moses; when he had not the energy to continue on in the desert, falling by a well, the unknown spirit pushed on.

On September 29, 2015, I did just that, made an appointment to see my personal doctor, the following day. That night, before my doctor's appointment, my feet had swollen badly, pain beyond understanding engulf my wellbeing. I tried to soak in Epson salt, thinking it may reduce the swelling and easy the pain, not so. Grandma always said, when faced with no other option take matters into your own hands, well with the pain increasing and no other options, I did just that, I cut a slight hole under the bottom of my foot to release pressure, low and behold; a gassy, bubbly substance, having a very terrible smell comes shooting out, hooray temporary relief. I got out of the tub, dried off and began preparing for bed. Shortly; upon entering bed, I began running a very high fever and just couldn't sleep again, I cut made another incision to relieve pressure, should not have done that, I thought to myself as blood began to oohs out. I did not sleep the entire night, starting upstairs and leaving a blood trail down into the family room, it was as my mother describe : as if a bomb went off in the house, everything turn upside down and out of place, blood everywhere as if soldiers had been on the battlefield and were quickly remove with no time to clear the aftermath of war. No choice but to stick it out until the morning, once again pride set in. As the sun began to rise in the eastern sky, I remembered: today is the day, which was September 30th. That morning was like no other and having not slept and no energy, I began to notice a dramatic change with regards to my body temperature and energy, could not walk two steps without gasping for air, shivering or having to seat down just to keep from fainting. Deciding it would be wise to get some quick burst of energy, I drove to MacDonald's and ordered a large O.J…O.J. why, in denial again, but for some reason I did not immediately drink, instead I waited until arriving in the parking lot of hospital to drink, which gave me enough energy to walk from parking lot into my doctor's office. After checking in, I sat down and my body started shaking uncontrollably, again I gather myself and proceeded to respond with all the procedures prior to seeing the doctor. Nurse Amy led me into the office and laid me down on a small bed. I curled up like a small child waiting for his/her parents alone and frightened. Alex he said, what's going on, immediately I took off my left shoe and exposed the wounded foot, seeing the look of great concern on his face,

I share the ordeal, my primary physician quickly called over to podiatry and Dr. Foot Specialist came right over, bit of luck that day, as usually a secondary appointment is needed, hooray! He began to examine and prod into my foot asking, whether I had feeling and my response was yes, I could feel all that was being done. He seems somewhat confused, as from a professional view, there was no chance in (the hottest place) of feeling. He ask me to close my eyes and again ask, if I could feel his prodding and again my answer was, yes. Then with a stern voice he commanded, open your eyes, to my amazement, they were both standing across the room gazing upon me. I thought for a moment, and said nothing. Dr. foot than came over and said to me, at this point I am not sure whether it will be your foot or your leg. I am leaving you to imagine for yourselves, the feeling that overcame me. They said, we need blood work to determine what else could be going on within the body. I was ask if I needed a wheelchair, as a soldier on the battlefield wounded, yet with the courage to continue, I strapped up my laces and walked to the lab. Moments later was immediately admitted into the hospital. I began to think: how did I get here, what did I do in life to deserve this. I was always the one willing to help, always with my hand on someone else, say it will be alright. Now, I need someone to do the same for me. I did I ever get a response. My mother, sisters and cousins, where there and their hand were on my shoulder. Again, I am trying to get away and in denial I ask, could I go home and come back, surgery would be another 4 hour due to consumption, the O.J. They answered no and I had emergency surgery to amputate half my left foot. The doctors who performed the surgery said; had I not come in that day, I would have lost my life before the sun rose the next morning. I was quite fortunate, as I had developed gas gangrene in my foot and it was infiltrating into my system, leading to septic shock which I was experiencing. The surgery was a success, only half my foot was amputated and not the entire leg. This was a major physiological victory which allowed me to deal with the lost.

In the hospital, dealing with the loss, erratic sugar levels, ego and my foolhardiness. Eight days later, I was transported home in a wheelchair, missing half my left foot or what they call a below ankle amputation. Daily I had nurses in and out attending to my health needs, bandage replacement on foot, which lasted 10 months. My family and I immediately went to work on curing sugar level and getting the right foods. It has been months since my surgery, with many more visits to podiatry, fitting for shoes, followed by intense therapy to regain quality of life skills and having dedicated myself to maintaining healthy sugar levels within the body through a change in diet and increased exercise, which effectively saw an A1C fall from 10.3 to 6.3 in one month and maintaining a normal level of 5.7 since. Not to say, I have not struggled with it from time to time.

Since being on the road to recovery, my physical pain had come to a halt, then came the emotional pain of wondering why me and never imaging going through life not able to do the things I was used to doing, such as, running, playing pickup game of basketball or dancing the night away, in the comfort of my home with my two daughters. I look out the window and saw so many who were suffering along with me, but had given up on themselves and life all together. Their questions not answered, and no one to help them on the long journey home. Although, I had a support system to get me through what I call phase 1, now I was getting ready for phase 2.

Phase 2

When the lights go out and the room becomes dark, I alone sat to ponder my next move. Would I fall back into my old ways or would I continue on the path I had set? It became a mental challenge, as the physical body started to exert its will upon me, calling for the bad foods which caused me so much pain and suffering. Calling for soda, sugars and preservatives to reenter and cause havoc. Many in my camp were skeptical about my determination and drive; they were saying under their breath, he will return to the bad habits once a sense of normality sets in. On these lonely nights, I kept reminding myself of what I had just gone through, time and time again, glancing at the left foot to keep me honest. Before the walls could close in and, before I fell back into old habits, just as a career criminal, not having the will or the desire to reframe from those bad intentions, always being pulled back in by fate or friends in the same circle, I turn to a higher source, a power that I knew from time. Making peace with what had happened and accepting there was something I could offer to others in place of bad intentions. We all are face with certain challenges in life, what we do in that time, will define our character; I want my definition to have a greater meaning, not to be a criminal falling back in crime and blaming society for ones entire shortcoming. I began to speak to people, about the need to be conscious of what they put into their bodies. I pointed out how the food and drug administration share the same office and how one hand wipes the other. Having a renewed purpose, I push back against my body needs, craving and wants before those walls, but as I turned the corner, a test must come ones way to determine, the true character of a person. Phase 3 began; this phase is known as setbacks

Phase 3

I believe one does not receive more than one can handle and at times a test is thrown at you; to challenge mental toughness and how one handle adversity. Well, I can honestly say, in the beginning it did not go well, but as Moses falling from Prince of Egypt, to wander the desert, not knowing destiny and conquering the conqueror, set forth beyond his comprehension, I felt that sense of what he was thinking, why me, why so much pain and so little reward for changing a way of life. I use Moses as a metaphor only in slight comparison as I could not walk in his shoes, but had a sense of the feeling. One day I am walking, running and dancing on top of my world, next day confined to a bed with no ability to walk, run or dance, yet there was a force behind pushing me on, no letup, no surrender and no quitting. My foot was healing incredibly well, doctors where amazed with the process, as many in position had a much longer time getting there. All could not have been going better, my family coming up on the weekends, house full of people, good food great times. Well, one Sunday afternoon while I sat on the couch watching the Raiders game, my daughter happen to walk by and noticed something unusual, she ask me for my ip-phone and took a picture. Weeks have passed; Constance glancing at the foot, making sure all is well, no signs to report, what was a healthy foot, change to an open wound with discoloration and built up fluid. Days after no sign of healing, I found myself back in the emergency room waiting and wondering the worse. Yet, the worse would not be on this day, after extensive testing, it was determine although had built up, there was no infection on the bones. Fluid as explained by the medical doctors, developed after 9 months of no activity and suddenly walking in excess, causing water to build at the base finding exit points, it made sense as gravity pulls down on all things. So now, I am once again back on the couch in bandages, another three weeks in order to allow the natural process of healing to run its course. Onward to my next destiny, the return phase 4 Back to Work

Phase 4

The return: The last time I thought about getting out in traffic, not moving for hours listening to horns, screeching tires and smell of vapors, a year ago just before going out on disability. One misses the friends and good time between employees and the special bonds we have with them, missed talking sports and politics. Meeting new customers and listening to their every need as a company and ability to offer solutions that impacts there bottom line. Most of what I missed was the smiles on the faces of satisfied customers, the joy it brought me knowing I had done my job well. Having said all that, the mind as it does, wondered, what life on the job would be like now. I am in pain and the swelling shows no sign of letting up, walking has become more of a burden than a right. How will I walk with my tools over shoulders and boxes in my hands? Since losing a good portion of my left foot, balance has become the number one concern. Over the course of a month I have adjusted accordingly, as the body does a good job of adapting to natural courses in life. I am very pleased with my progress at work, not taking on a workload beyond what I can handle and not over exhorting the body, mind and spirit. Upper management has been great, bringing me back slowly and not giving an over aggressive workload. I am looking to begin taking on more in six month. Half the year gone and workload has increased to a steady flow of issues to resolve. I am now closing out 2017; I can say, all went well on the home front. Foot held up just fine swelling subsided and walking became a non-issue. Thanks to all my fellow employees giving the support upon my return and assisting me when I call on them.

Phase 5

Life: we all can agree it is a struggle to continue to apply truth to most things in regards to health, as we are bombarded daily with TV ads and colors which attract the human mind to stand up, listening and watching attentively. This brings to me the last frontier on my long journey home, in keeping a healthy lifestyle. How will I counteract these ads without going into seclusion, should I not watch the local games on Sundays? Should I not look at billboards driving down the highway; can I listen to music without commercials of tasty foods and sodas that have been part of my childhood and adult life? How will I continue to eat correctly while working around so many unhealthy restaurants? Life has many curve balls to throw at us, still we must remind ourselves of the sacrifice which must be taken in order to continue living. Each and every day I am reminded of such, when looking down at my foot, as I ask the question: how much more? My answer; no more, this is it and with that said, "affirm life as it should be and not as it was". I am healthy enjoying my walks and getting to meet and share my experience with others, helping them, so that they will not have to endure the painful process. Having a second chance and using it to do the will of human-kindness. It is easier to go the negative route because there are so many avenues, and so few in the positive direction. When we accept the positive route as the norm, more doors open in greater areas as never before. I did not imagine writing a book, but here I am doing so, did not imagine speaking to people in hospitals and conferences, nor having an impact on so many, yet it did. I continue to push the doors of positive change in regards to health, as it is related to our overall being. So, help me by taking care of yourselves and remembering my ordeal, as you take the next 32 oz. soda or big gulp or down a greasy burger. I am not saying we can't have such; I am simply saying, eat healthier throughout the year and barbeque Super Bowl weekend and why shouldn't we? After all, eating health year round does give us liberty to cheat on the big holidays, wouldn't you agree! Thank you for reading and taking time to allow my story into your life, I hope it will have a lasting impact on you or a family member you have shared this with.

Shalom!

Diabetes the disease

I would like to briefly discuss what I have learned about: diabetes the disease and how a good diet plan will impact your health and ensure more years with love ones. Diabetes is a disease that works in the shadows, slowly unleashing itself within the body, attaching to cells and causing transmission signals along the central system. This disease has affected millions of people worldwide and growing, mostly due to improper diet. It has world health organization calling for countries to do a better job sounding the alarm. In the United States, it has become the fastest growing disease and health concern. Diabetes comes about when the pancreas does not produce enough insulin or properly regulate the insulin produced, resulting in high levels of sugar traveling within the body unregulated, which can cause issues to liver and kidney over time.

Question is why?

Over the years governments have been exploring ways to better feed their growing population in an effort to stop mass starvation. In doing so, a new sugar was develop which could be process quicker and cheaper than having to turn normal sugar into an unnatural form, as sugar is brown in color and then is bleached and enriched, the result white sugar. High fructose corn syrup was developed as a substitute. Since its development, countries have seen high level of their population become diabetic, especially children. What was not known up until recently, was the correlation between this synthetic sugar and the decease. Researchers and human rights groups began making the case: there is direct link, but food manufactures in their need to turn profits continued to ignore these groups, leading to the expansion of diabetes globally. Only after long battles with Americans for diabetes and advocacy groups, some manufactures began going back to traditional sugars.

There are two types of this disease: Type I, which is usually acquired from birth and Type 2 which has to do with diet, age and heredity.

Type 1

The more severe form of diabetes is insulin-dependent diabetes. It's sometimes called "juvenile" diabetes, because this type of diabetes usually develops in children and teenagers. If you are diagnose, you will have to take insulin and manage as a lifelong disease. We have no cure for this decease at the moment.

Type 2

Diabetes is a medical condition in which sugar, or glucose, levels build up in your bloodstream. There's not enough insulin made in pancreas to regulate the sugar cells thus causes your body to rely on alternative energy sources in your tissues, muscles, and organs, symptoms may be mild and easy to dismiss at first.

The early symptoms may include:

- constant hunger
- a lack of energy
- fatigue
- weight loss
- excessive thirst
- frequent urination
- dry mouth
- itchy skin
- blurry vision

All of which I experience but paid no mind, as the disease progresses, the symptoms become more severe and potentially dangerous. If undetected, blood sugar levels may become more aggressive and include:

- yeast infections
- slow-healing cuts or sores
- dark patches on your skin
- foot pain
- Feelings of numbness in your extremities, or neuropathy.

This can cause limbs to be amputated, as in my case. Diabetes has a powerful effect on your heart. So it is important to maintain blood pressure level of 120/70 and exercise 30 mins daily, to prevent heart attacks and strokes. Blood test can show level of sugar in system, one type of test call A1C, determines the average amount of sugar in your bloodstream over a ninety day period. This type of test is essential, as many can cheat with daily testing by exercising 20 minutes prior, causing sugar level to fall to acceptable measures.

Diet Plan

Diet is an important tool to combat diabetes, also keeping your heart healthy and strong. Diabetic people need to eat more fresh vegetables. It is very important to change your eating habits, i.e. food intake. It doesn't have to be complicated or unpleasant. The diet recommended for people with type 2 diabetes is the same diet just about everyone should follow; it boils down to dedication and commitment. A few key actions below:

- Eat meals and snacks on schedule.
- Choose a variety of foods that are high in nutrition and low in empty calories.
- Be careful not to overeat.
- Read food labels closely

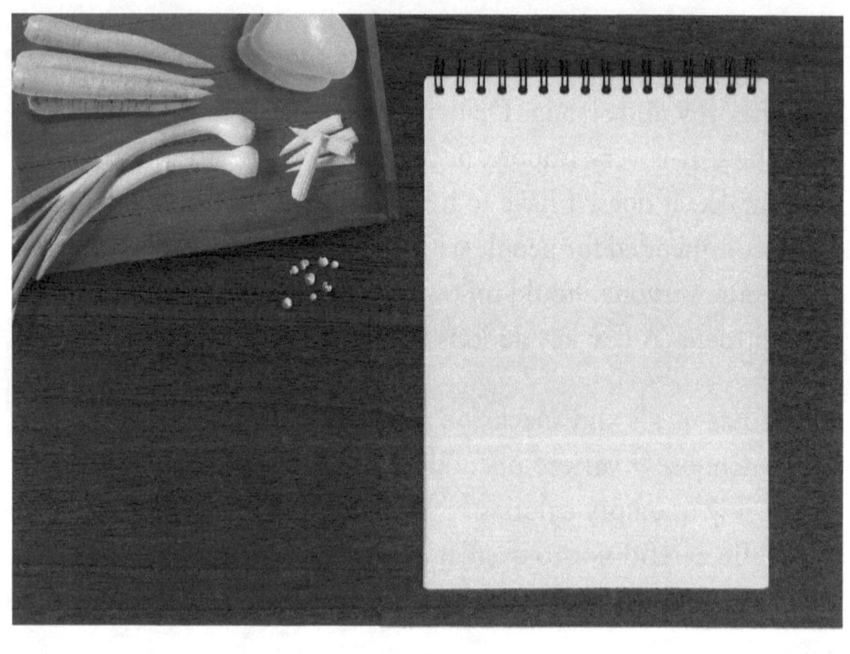

Foods to choose

Healthy carbohydrates can provide you with fiber. The options include:

- vegetables
- fruits
- legumes, such as beans
- whole grains

Foods with heart-healthy omega-3 fatty acids include:

- tuna
- sardines
- salmon
- mackerel
- halibut
- cod

You can get healthy fats from a number of foods other than meat, including:

- olive oil
- canola oil
- peanut oil

- almonds
- pecans
- walnuts
- avocados
- Beans

Although these options for fat are good, they're high in calories, moderation is key, choose low-fat options.

Foods to avoid

There are certain foods that you should limit or avoid entirely. These include:

- foods heavy in saturated fats
- foods heavy in trans fats
- beef
- processed meats
- shellfish
- stick margarine
- shortening
- baked goods
- processed snacks
- sugary drinks
- high-fat dairy products
- salty foods
- fried foods

Foods with Preservatives should be avoided when possible, through trial and error; I found hidden in those preservatives and not disclosed on labels, high amounts of sugar and unhealthy carbs. Companies are not required to reveal those ingredients.

With all diets one should consult a physician or dietitian before enacting on any such undertaking. I hope the information I have provided will help in aiding a healthy diet and life style. Remember there's nothing wrong with treating yourself every now and then to a nice meal, as we all need to enjoy some of life's fruits.

Recipes

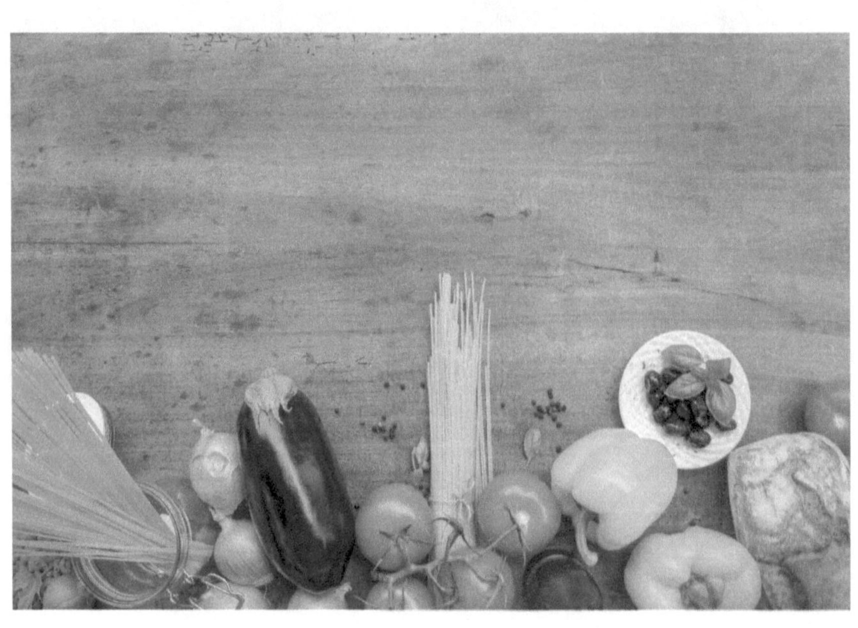

Creole Soup

Ingredients

2 zucchini Julian or chopped

3 medium onions

1 bunch asparagus chopped

2 shredded carrots

½ cabbages chopped

¼ cup of yogurt

1 can of garbanzo beans

2 cloves of garlic

1 tsp of turmeric

3 pinches Cayenne pepper

2 tsp of coconut oil

½ lb. of turkey ground

Preparation

Sauté all vegetables in coconut oil, add 1 teaspoon turmeric, salt and pepper until tender, add chicken stock and garbanzo beans, ¼ cup of yogurt

Shred ½ lb. chicken or ground turkey to vegetable, let cook for 15 to 20 minutes and serve.

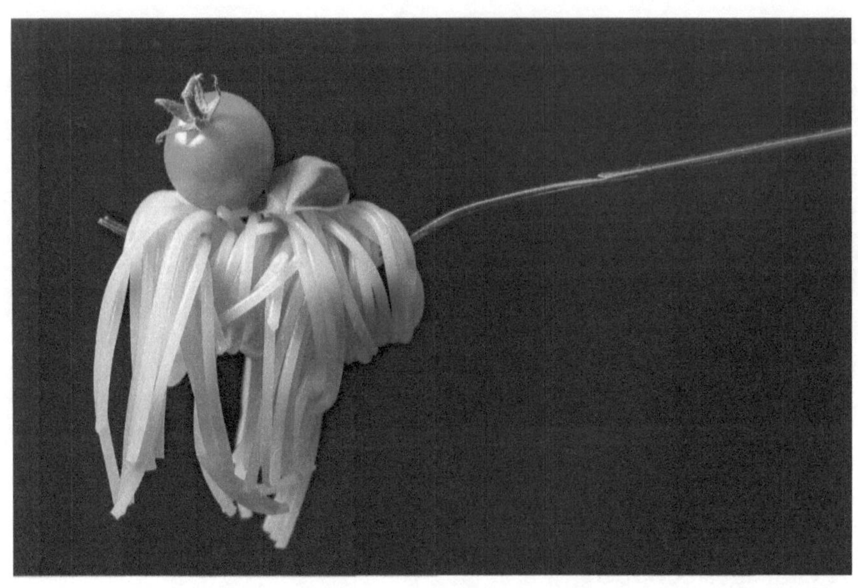

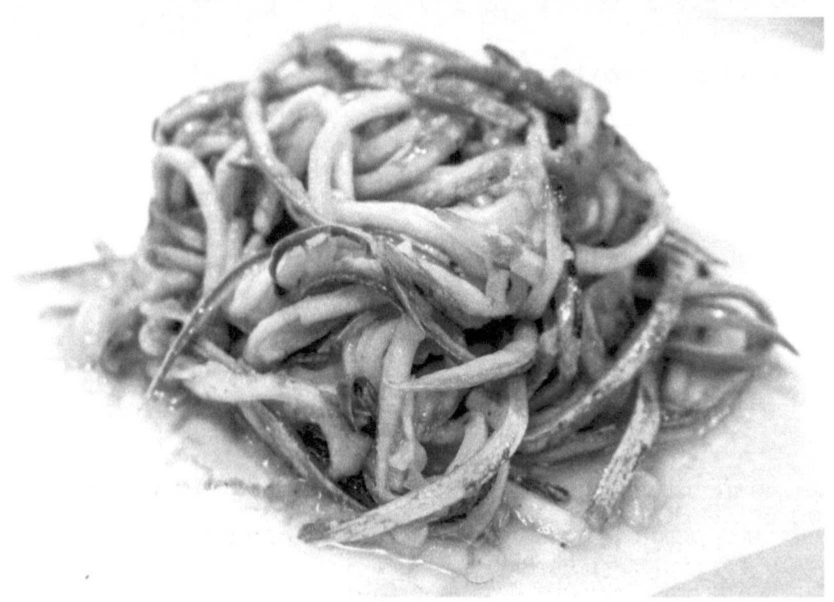

Stuffed Spaghetti Squash

Ingredients

1 spaghetti squash cut in half

3 tablespoon coconut oil

3 cups kale

3 cups spinach

1 small onion

3 cloves garlic

½ teaspoon saffron powder

½ green and red bell pepper

½ teaspoon harissa spices sugar free

½ teaspoon turmeric powder

1 cup Mexican four cheeses

1 teaspoon apple cider vinegar

Preparation

In a non-stick baking pan place slice halves squash side down, brush coconut oil inside the two halves and bake at 350 degrees for 20 to 25 minutes, remove from oven and set aside to cool.

In skillet: add 2 tablespoons of coconut oil, sauté onion, garlic, bell peppers after sauté add saffron powder, turmeric, salt and pepper, spinach and kale sauté 4 to 5 minutes.

Using a fork, scrape out the flesh of halves squash and add to sauté pan, mix gently all ingredients with 1/2 of Mexican cheese. After mixing, distribute into squash halves shells. Top off with remainder of cheese and bake at 350 degrees for 20 to 30 mins.

Enjoy a remarkable lunch or dinner time meal that will open your taste buds and have all talking at the table.

Kidney Bean Salad

Ingredients

1 can kidney bean

½ red bell pepper chopped

1 medium tomato chopped

1 small red onion chopped

½ lemon squeezed

3 tablespoon olive oil

2 tablespoon parsley

Preparation

Mix ingredients together, add salt and pepper at your leisure. I recommend without salt. Now enjoy a nice night time light salad not heavy on the stomach but filling and healthy.

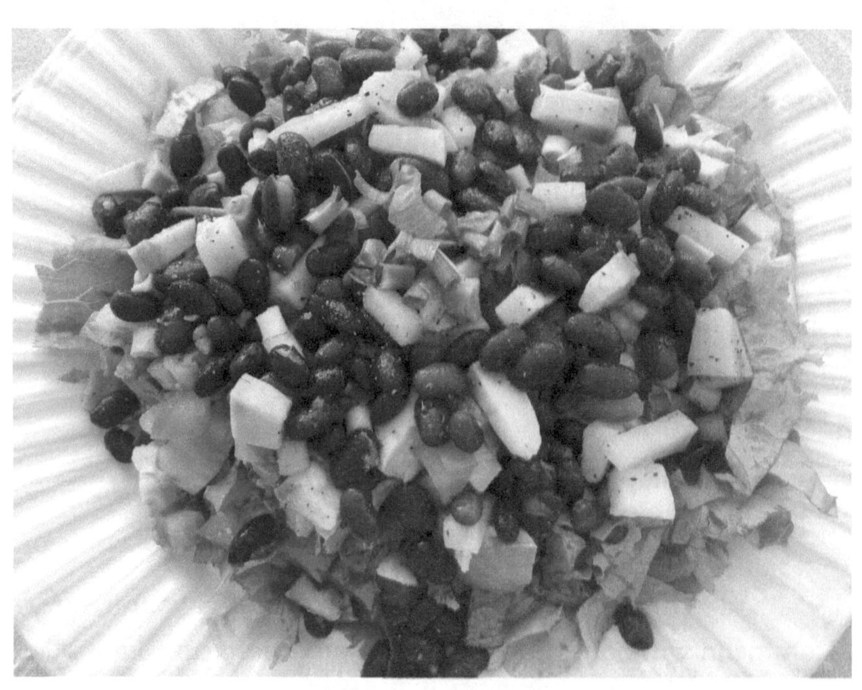

Black Bean Stir Fry Salad

Ingredients
1 can black bean
½ red and green bell pepper chopped
1 medium tomato chopped
1 red onion chopped
1 lemon
2 tablespoons oil or olive oil
1 avocado

<u>Stir fry</u>
1 cup quinoa
1 onion
3 cloves garlic
2 celery sticks
¾ lb. turkey meat
½ lemon zest
½ cup white wine
1 teaspoon turmeric
1 cup carrot chopped
3 cups kale
3 cups spinach

Preparation

Cook 1 cup quinoas in 1 cup of water bring to a boil, turn down and allow steaming 15mins

In a separate pan cook ¾ turkey meat with onions and garlic until brown, add vegetables, salt and pepper to taste

Open can black bean drain and wash

Wash all ingredients prior to mixing

Put in bowl and mix in all other ingredients,

In a plate; pour cooked turkey and vegetables over quinoa add black bean salad, cut 2 slices of avocado and serve.

I am writing this book as it relates to my actual experience, that is why it is important to keep it as is. People want to read not at length ones ordeal, but how it impact their lives and what was done to recover. Many are waiting to read; from the doctors who treated me to the many that I have come in contact with. They all are eager to share with member of their family, who are currently struggling with diabetes and the many patients who can benefit from what I did to turn it all around within a year. So remember, it is not the quantity of words, but the quality of words in life.

Thank you
Alexander Danny Joyeux